INTERMITTENT FASTING FOR WOMEN OVER 30

A FREAKISHLY SIMPLE GUIDE TO LOSING UP TO 15 LBS IN 30 DAYS WITHOUT GOING TO THE GYM

I.J. RODZ

This is for all women who wish to lose weight but with everything going on in their lives it is hard to even think about it. For all the women who wish to wear those pre-pregnancy jeans when they lose that baby weight. For all the women who have been criticized because of how they look. For all the women who feel self-conscious after pregnancy. For all the women to start respecting and loving themselves once again.

- I.J. Rodz

INTRODUCTION

Hi! My name is I.J. Rodz. I've always been overweight since I can remember. When I was 9 years old, I was weighing 125 lbs. Some kids in school would call me "free Willy" (by then the movie had just come out). It made me feel self-conscious and with many insecurities.

That frustrated me. I loved food of any kind and I wanted to eat it. It was something I couldn't resist. I am from Puerto Rico and most of the typical foods we eat are fried, sweet bread, rice, and beans, homemade sweets, etc. Puertorican food taste so good with really good spices.

Growing up in the 90s there wasn't enough education about how to eat a balanced meal. I remember my grandma would tell me that I need to eat because if I don't I get weak. Sometimes if I didn't eat all of the food on my plate I couldn't go outside to play with my cousins.

During my pre-teenage years, I wanted to wear fashionable clothes. My sister was the skinny type and she always eat whatever and never gain weight. I always wanted to wear her clothes but they never fit me. So I had to wear baggy clothes because my dad said I was too voluptuous at my age and didn't want any guy looking at me. Now, I'm ok with that because I have kids but back then I would get mad. I couldn't wear trendy clothes because of how big I was.

Anyways, forwarding a few years when I was in high school, I was able to drop about 15 pounds just by running a few laps around the apartment complex we used to live in. Even though my sister's clothes didn't fit me yet, I could wear some trendy clothes with my nice curves. I was very happy. Then, in college, I gained all the weight again. I guess it was from all the stress with so many assignments. Or maybe it was so many Chipotle burritos I ate every day (laughing).

A few years later I got married, gave birth to my first child, and bada bing bada boom I was weighing 190 lbs. I was a size 14 in clothes. Never in my life have I weighed so much. I didn't want to buy new clothes because I knew I was going to lose weight. I started exercising and using a point system and was able to lose 30 pounds. But I stopped exercising and stopped paying for the point system and slowly was gaining it all back.

Three years passed, and got pregnant again. Gave birth. I weighed myself on the scale and was almost 200 lbs. I kept wearing my maternity clothes. I didn't even want to take pictures of myself. I was very self-conscious about myself again. This time my friend told me about a program where you follow an eating plan and you could include the Spanish foods that you like. So I started it and did lose 30 pounds in about a year. Then a hurricane passed by Florida (where I currently live) and I had to go back to eating bad food since we were without electricity for about 2 weeks. I didn't follow the plan anymore and gained it all back.

After this, I wanted to give up. I didn't care anymore if I was overweight. Just kept my bad ways of eating unbalanced meals at whatever time of day. I was eating all the leftovers from my children's food. I felt bad throwing them away. My meals were not balanced either. I did not want to exercise. I needed to lay down on my bed at noon to take a nap because I didn't have any energy at all.

Then, one day, as I was scrolling through my Instagram and saw a video of someone talking about how her health got better and how fit she was because she started intermittent fasting and eating a high-fat diet. My mind thought... "What? She starved herself and only ate fats?

Gosh! That's why I am overweight because of my excessive fat. Why would I want to eat it?"

I learned to be always open-minded and humbled to be able to learn new things. So I started researching intermittent fasting and high-fat diets. Surprisingly, it wasn't what I thought it was. I learned all the health benefits of doing both and how you could prevent many diseases while at the same time losing weight.

So I found the book about intermittent fasting by Dr. Jason Fung. Wow, such a learning experience. Just reading it gave me the chills thinking how I have never heard of this before. I am glad it came at the right time just exactly when I needed it.

In this book, this is what I will tell you. Exactly what I followed to lose 15 lbs in 1 month. By the time I am writing this book it already has been 30 pounds and counting. It feels great to fit in a size 10 again and wear trendy clothes whenever I want to.

You must know that I am not a nutritionist or doctor. This is all information from what I learned and applied. I always advice people to consult their doctor first about starting a new diet.

When you start implementing this challenge into your life, you will feel so much better. I can assure you it will be something that you can carry over for the rest of your life without bouncing back to where you were.

In this 30-day challenge, you will learn...

What foods to avoid forever!!!

 What fats are the ones keeping you fat?

 The carbohydrates that make you gain even though you thought they were healthy

 What times of day to eat

 Why is intermittent fasting so important

 How to keep off that weight to never bounce back

 How to follow an eating plan to make it a lifestyle

In the next chapter, you will learn why fats are important to consume plus a shopping list to make that pantry look so much healthier and your fridge too.

A MAKEOVER FOR YOUR PANTRY AND FRIDGE

$\mathcal{I}$ remember in the 90s there were TV commercials talking about how fat was so bad for you. It was the reason you were fat according to them. Most of the food was advertised as low fat or zero trans fat.

Well, I have good news for you. Fat is a necessary macronutrient for your body to function especially for your body to create energy. However, there is always a catch. There is good fat and bad fat. The bad fats are trans fats. Why are they bad? Because they have been processed by adding hydrogen to vegetable oils to make them into solids and to have a longer shelf life. Trans fat is usually found in heavily processed foods. On the other hand, there are good fats that your body needs. Monosaturated fats help reduce your LDL levels (bad cholesterol) such as olive oil. Polyunsaturated fats like omega 3 and 6 help your nervous system function better.

Fats give the body the energy it needs so your body can function the way it should. During exercise, your body uses the calories from carbohydrates you have consumed. After 20 minutes your body has consumed all calories from carbohydrates. Then, your body will use the calories from the fat you have consumed so you can keep going. Believe it or not, it helps your body keep warm, and for your brain to function well your need fats.

Surprisingly, your body needs fats so your skin and hair look healthy. Liposoluble vitamins such as A, D, E, and K are absorbed better with the help of fats. Our body needs other nutrients protein and carbohydrates. We need proteins to build strong muscles and bones, regulate hormones and keep our immune system strong. Carbohydrates are the body's nutrients for energy.

For these 30 days, your plate will have 5% carbohydrates, 25% protein, and 70% fats. You will notice how great fats are for your body.

In this challenge, you will eat more fats than protein or carbohydrates. Prepare your mind from now on to stop eating sugar. By sugar, I mean everything that your body can process as sugar.

Don't worry, here is the list:

- Sugar
- Bread (any kind)
- Vegetable roots (potatoes, beets, carrots, etc)
- Alcoholic drinks
- Juices of any kind

- Fruits
- Beans of any kind
- Corn
- Green beans
- Peanuts
- Rice
- Plantain
- Beets
- Red, orange, and yellow peppers
- Sweet potato
- Radishes
- sweets

Fats to avoid:

- Canola oil
- Soy oil
- Sunflower oil
- Grape seed oil
- Corn oil

No Flours of any kind:

- Corn flour
- Wheat flour
- Coconut flour
- Almond flour
- No flaxseed flour
- No oatmeal flour

- No popcorn

Vegetables to avoid

- Cucumber (not many nutrients, fiber, or carbs)
- Lettuce (not many nutrients, fiber, or carbs)

Here is a list of approved vegetables. These are good carbohydrates. Choose the one you like the most. Have an open mind about eating them. These are very healthy and will take you closer to your weight loss goal.

Shopping list for Approved Vegetables:

- Spinach
- Arugula
- Chard
- Bok choy
- Celery
- Cauliflower
- Zucchini
- Cabbage
- Kale
- Broccoli
- Asparagus
- Brussel sprouts
- Artichoke
- Celery
- Mushrooms
- Eggplant

This is your shopping list for approved animal proteins. Choose the ones you will eat and have an open mind about which ones you want to try:

Approved animal proteins

- Beef
- Turkey
- Salmon
- Pork
- Chicken
- Cows belly
- Liver
- Lobster
- Eggs
- Shrimp
- Mussels
- Bacon
- Lamb
- Tuna
- Fish
- eggs

Here is your shopping list for healthy approved fats:

- Avocado
- Mayonnaise
- Bacon
- Walnuts
- Pork rinds (plain, no flavor)

- Almonds
- Green olives
- Cheese
- Salmon
- Cream cheese
- Sour cream
- MCT Oil
- Extra virgin Olive oil
- Avocado Oil
- Coconut oil

Miscellaneous Items you will need:

- Apple cider vinegar (with the mother raw unfiltered)
- Baking soda
- Sea salt
- Himalayan salt
- Matcha powder (0 carbs no sugar)
- green tea

Have fun buying your food items. If you are not used to eating those items, don't worry you will start to love them. Especially after you see the pounds coming off the scale. Now moving to the next chapter which is portion control.

YOUR HANDS CONTROL WHAT
YOU EAT

*H*ere, I will show you how to use your hands to measure the portions of fats, carbohydrates, and animal proteins you put on your plate. Note this step is very important because if you put more or less than what I show you here, your body will be getting not enough or too much of what you eat. If you use more, then your body can use it as more energy than it needs. That means more accumulated fat than you want to. If you are not putting enough then your body will not function as it should.

There are different portions for women and men. Since men have more mass and are usually bigger than women, they need more to eat. Please women, no matter how hungry you feel after eating your portions don't think following the men's portions is better. Men, please don't think it's OK to eat more than your regular portion sizes. This will affect your results.Portion sizes for women

. . .

THIS IS how you measure animal proteins with your hand:

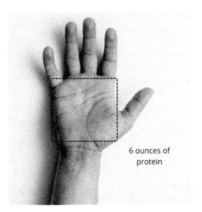

6 ounces of
protein

THIS IS how you measure animal protein for women that is hard to measure with hands:

- Chicken drumsticks: 2 chicken drumsticks
- Eggs: 2 whole eggs with egg yolk
- Tuna: 1 can of tuna
- Shrimp- 8-10 shrimps

THIS IS how you measure vegetables with your hand for women:

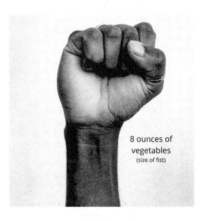

8 ounces of
vegetables
(size of fist)

THIS IS how you measure fats:

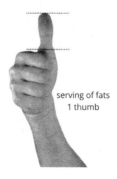

serving of fats
1 thumb

PORTION SIZES for men

THIS IS how you measure animal proteins for men:

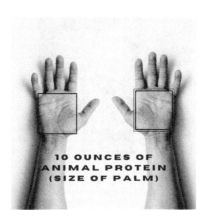

FOR MEN, Animal protein that it is hard to measure with hands, you will measure it like this:

- Chicken drumstick (with skin)- for men 3 drumsticks
- Eggs (whole)- 3 eggs with yolk
- Tuna- 200 grams of tuna
- Shrimp- 12 shrimps

THIS IS how you measure vegetables for men:

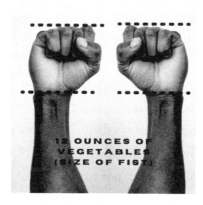

THIS IS how you measure fat (same for men and woman):

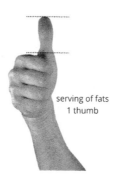

THESE ARE examples of portion fat sizes per meal. Choose only one per meal:

- Avocado: ½ avocado per meal (1 whole avocado a day)
- Mayonnaise: 2 tbsp per meal
- Bacon: only 2 slices
- Pork rinds (plain no flavor): 4-6 pork rinds
- Almonds: 8-9 almonds
- Green olives: 8-10 per meal
- Cheese: the size of 2 fingers
- Salmon: if you eat salmon, don't need to add fat
- Cream cheese: 2 tbsp
- Sour cream: 2 tbsp

IF YOU WANT to measure your food in volumes these are the portion sizes for men and women:

TYPE OF FOOD
    Men
    Women
    Animal protein
    10 oz/ 284 gr/ 296ml
    6 oz/ 170 gm/ 178 ml
    Vegetables

12 oz/ 340 gm/ 355 ml

8 oz/ 226 gm/ 236 ml

Fats

1 thumb size

1 thumb size

IN THE NEXT Chapter you'll know everything about fasting. You will start to get a sense of what this 30 days will be all about.

WHAT YOU DIDN'T KNOW ABOUT FASTING

*B*efore I ever knew about the benefits of fasting, I thought people were crazy. I mean why people are starving themselves? I can't do that. If I fast, I will faint before noon.

That was my mentality about fasting. As time passed, I heard people getting results from doing this not only losing weight but having more energy and their health getting better.

When I started reading the book, The Complete Guide to Fasting by Jason Fung, I was so surprised. This guy would go for weeks fasting just to know how his body responded to it. As he kept doing this, he realized the less he craved food. I think it was amazing.

So the more I read the more I learned and wanted to try it as well. So there are different times that you can fast. For beginners, you should start no more than 14 hours. After you are used to this and your body feels accustomed to it, you can start increasing the fasting hours, to 16, 18, or 24 hours.

Don't worry if you are starting we will start at 14 hours. I thought I couldn't do it at first but surprisingly I felt awesome. I will show you how you can trick your body to stay in fasting mode while giving the nutrients it needs so you don't feel like you are starving yourself.

So let's begin...

What is Intermittent Fasting?

This is restricted eating where you have only a certain amount of eating window. For example, you can fast for 16 hours a day and eat 8 hours a day. When I say to eat 8 hours a day, I don't mean you will continuously eat for 8 hours. No. What I mean is, you can have 2-3 balanced meals during those 8 hours.

This method is most popular because people fast while sleeping at night, it is just a few hours where we don't actually eat while awake. For example, your last meal is at 8 pm, then you sleep the next day until 6 am. You could eat your first meal at 12 pm. This will make 16 hours of fasting. Now from 12 to 8 pm you could have 2-3 meals (2.5 hours between every meal). Then repeat the next day. There are other times of fasting like 14/10, 18/6, or 24-hour fasting.

So you may ask, what happens to our body when we fast? Our body gets clean from toxins and our cells start working much better because it forces our body to get energy from other means and materials. When we fast, our body doesn't get the energy from what we eat but from the fat that is stored in our body. No wonder we lose weight!

Benefits of fasting

- Makes your brain works better
- Protect you from becoming obese
- Reduces inflammation
- You will get fit
- Support losing weight
- Prevents metabolic diseases

When you fast for more than 16 hours, your body goes into a process called autophagy where your cells start to regenerate which destroys old damaged cells in the body. When you start this you will feel weird and is good to know what to do and what things to look for. Here is a list of things you can feel when you start fasting:

- You will feel hungry and fatigued because the body feels low from energy and glucose
- You can feel tired
- You can have leg cramps (don't worry I tell you how to prevent them from happening)
- Glucogenesis will start to occur when your body will start to get the energy from the fat in your body (weight loss)
- Gradually your body will get used to fasting and you won't feel hungry
- Having a healthy meal after fasting increases

insulin sensitivity which helps in fat loss and
helps the body prevent diseases such as
diabetes, high blood pressure and heart diseases

Fasting concerns

Hunger: it is normal you could feel this way compared to the way you were eating. Try to stay busy. You won't feel hungry all the time. As your body gets used to fasting, it will start using the stores of fat for energy so hunger will start to decrease. Drink water, coffee, green tea and add a dash of cinnamon (it also helps to decrease hunger).

Dizziness: If you feel dizzy, you most probably are dehydrated. You can add himalayan salt to your water. It will help. Be sure to drink plenty of liquids.

Headaches: it is normal if you feel headaches. Transitioning from eating foods with salt to low salt intake during fasting it could happen. Know they will disappear in time. In the mean time, put a tsp of himalayan salt in water and it will help.

Constipation: It is normal and expected. This is because you are eating less food and fasting for longer periods. Make sure you are eating your vegetables during your meals.

Heartburn: avoid eating a big meal after a fast. Avoid lying down in bed after eating. Sparkling water with lemon can help. If you don't have sparkling water, Just add 1 tsp of baking soda to 16 oz of water and squeeze one whole lemon and drink. If it persists, consult your physician.

Muscle cramps: This means you need Magnesium. Drink Magnesium supplements.

The bottom line, fasting is a powerful tool to make you live longer and transform your health. You will see great results with this 30-day challenge.

SUPPLEMENTS ARE A MUST!!!

*S*ince most of the food we eat is cooked and processed, most of the nutrients it comes with are gone. That's why supplements are so important.

These will be your supplements for the next 30 days and if you decide to continue with this lifestyle you will need to get used to them. Along with the supplement, I have included a link or a QR code that will take you to the ones I recommend to buy on amazon that way it is easier for you to find. Just open your phone's camera and scan it. Then click the link it comes up.

Make sure these supplements don't include any of these ingredients:

- Stevia
- Sucralose
- Soybean oil

- Rice flour
- Maltodextrin
- Soy protein
- Xylitol
- Sorbitol
- No flavors of any kind
- Sunflower oil
- Safflower oil
- No gummies (it has sugar)
- Dextrose
- Sorbitol
- Lactose

HERE ARE the supplements you will need:

POTASSIUM GLUCONATE: Make sure it says Potassium gluconate https://amzn.to/38WfZg7

BIOTIN HTTPS://AMZN.TO/3LQuKI1

B12 HTTPS://AMZN.TO/3A0LCUI

COLLAGEN (NO FLAVOR) powder or pills https://www.4life.com/9794557/product/4life-transfer-factor-collagen-type-i/2409

https://amzn.to/3wXVGIw

MAGNESIUM GLUCONATE OR CITRATE HTTPS://AMZN.TO/ 3NKGUIZ

DAYS 1-10

*F*inally finally! Let's start the challenge. These 10 days are nothing like you have ever experienced. I will warn you that you will feel different. Remember you are getting sugar off your body for these next 30 days. A detox. You will be fine. It is the start of something great in your life and the starting path to a better you.

For these next 10 days, you will follow the 14/10 fasting period (14 hours fasting and 10 hours of eating period. This is a great way to start any fasting if you are a beginner. You won't feel it much since most of your fasting will be while you sleep.

These times you can accommodate to your schedule depending on what time you wake up or go to bed. Just make sure you are fasting for 14 hours and eating for 10 hours. You got this!

It is highly recommended you include at least 30 minutes of exercise every day. I suggest walking for 30 minutes. If you don't want to get out of your house you can go to youtube and find walking-in place videos for 30 minutes. It could be cardio for beginners for 30 minutes. When you include exercise your results will be faster and your body will use more energy to burn fat.

On your first day when you wake up, it is a must to weigh yourself. After you do that, grab a measuring tape and measure your body parts. Bellow, write down your starting weight and measurements.

DATE:_____
   Starting weight:_____

BODY MEASUREMENTS:

BICEPS L/R:_____
   Bust:_____
   Waist:_____ .
   Hip: _____
   Thighs L/R:_____

TWO RECIPES you need to know and do before you start. These two are the morning tea with apple cider vinegar and your morning special coffee. Don't worry they are easy to make. Here they are:

Apple cider vinegar morning tea Ingredients:

- 1 cup of warm water
- ½ lemon
- 1 tbsp of apple cider vinegar

How to prepare:

In one cup (8oz) of warm water, squeeze ½ lemon and pour 1 tbsp of apple cider vinegar, and stir. Use a straw to drink

Morning coffee ingredients: (this will keep you fasting)

- Brewed hot coffee
- 1 tbsp of MCT Oil (You can get this one at Amazon, Walmart, or any supermarket

How to prepare:

In a blender, pour 8 oz of hot coffee and MCT oil. Blend for 10 seconds. Pour in mug and drink

Bulletproof coffee ingredients:

- Hot brewed coffee (no flavor)
- 1 tbsp of MCT oil
- 1 tsp of stick butter
- 2 tbsp of half and half
- Collagen powder

How to prepare:

In a blender, blend coffee, MCT oil, butter, half and half, and collagen powder. Pour it into a mug and enjoy!

DAY 1:

- 7 am: drink apple cider vinegar tea
- Wait for 30 minutes
- 7:30 drink morning coffee
- 11:00: pm eat your first meal with protein, carbohydrates, and fats
- Soon after that drink your potassium, b12, and biotin
- 4 pm: eat your second meal with protein, carbohydrates, and fats
- After you eat your food drink your magnesium (before 5 pm)
- 9 pm drink your bulletproof coffee with collagen
- If collagen is powder put it inside coffee. If they are on pills drink them before coffee.
- after the bulletproof coffee, you can only drink water until the next day
- 30-minute simple exercise

DAY 2:

- 7 am: drink apple cider vinegar tea
- Wait for 30 minutes
- 7:30 drink morning coffee
- 11:00: pm eat your first meal with protein, carbohydrates, and fats
- Soon after that drink your potassium, b12, and biotin
- 4 pm: eat your second meal with protein, carbohydrates, and fats
- After you eat your food drink your magnesium (before 5 pm)
- 9 pm drink your bulletproof coffee with collagen
- If collagen is powder put it inside coffee. If they are on pills drink them before coffee.
- After the bulletproof coffee, you can only drink water until the next day
- 30-minute simple exercise

DAY 3:

- 7 am: drink apple cider vinegar tea
- Wait for 30 minutes
- 7:30 drink morning coffee

- 11:00: pm eat your first meal with protein, carbohydrates, and fats
- Soon after that drink your potassium, b12, and biotin
- 4 pm: eat your second meal with protein, carbohydrates, and fats
- After you eat your food drink your magnesium (before 5 pm)
- 9 pm drink your bulletproof coffee with collagen
- If collagen is powder put it inside coffee. If they are on pills drink them before coffee.
- After the bulletproof coffee, you can only drink water until the next day
- 30-minute simple exercise

DAY 4:

- 7 am: drink apple cider vinegar tea
- Wait for 30 minutes
- 7:30 drink morning coffee
- 11:00: pm eat your first meal with protein, carbohydrates, and fats
- Soon after that drink your potassium, b12, and biotin
- 4 pm: eat your second meal with protein, carbohydrates, and fats

- After you eat your food drink your magnesium (before 5 pm)
- 9 pm drink your bulletproof coffee with collagen
- If collagen is powder put it inside coffee. If they are on pills drink them before coffee.
- After the bulletproof coffee, you can only drink water until the next day
- 30-minute simple exercise

DAY 5:

- 7 am: drink apple cider vinegar tea
- Wait for 30 minutes
- 7:30 drink morning coffee
- 11:00: pm eat your first meal with protein, carbohydrates, and fats
- Soon after that drink your potassium, b12, and biotin
- 4 pm: eat your second meal with protein, carbohydrates, and fats
- After you eat your food drink your magnesium (before 5 pm)
- 9 pm drink your bulletproof coffee with collagen
- If collagen is powder put it inside coffee. If they are on pills drink them before coffee.

- After the bulletproof coffee, you can only drink water until the next day
- 30-minute simple exercise

Day 6:

- 7 am: drink apple cider vinegar tea
- Wait for 30 minutes
- 7:30 drink morning coffee
- 11:00: pm eat your first meal with protein, carbohydrates, and fats
- Soon after that drink your potassium, b12, and biotin
- 4 pm: eat your second meal with protein, carbohydrates, and fats
- After you eat your food drink your magnesium (before 5 pm)
- 9 pm drink your bulletproof coffee with collagen
- If collagen is powder put it inside coffee. If they are on pills drink them before coffee.
- After the bulletproof coffee, you can only drink water until the next day
- 30-minute simple exercise

Day 7:

- 7 am: drink apple cider vinegar tea
- Wait for 30 minutes
- 7:30 drink morning coffee
- 11:00: pm eat your first meal with protein, carbohydrates, and fats
- Soon after that drink your potassium, b12, and biotin
- 4 pm: eat your second meal with protein, carbohydrates, and fats
- After you eat your food drink your magnesium (before 5 pm)
- 9 pm drink your bulletproof coffee with collagen
- If collagen is powder put it inside coffee. If they are on pills drink them before coffee.
- After the bulletproof coffee, you can only drink water until the next day
- 30-minute simple exercise

Day 8:

- 7 am: drink apple cider vinegar tea
- Wait for 30 minutes
- 7:30 drink morning coffee

- 11:00: pm eat your first meal with protein, carbohydrates, and fats
- Soon after that drink your potassium, b12, and biotin
- 4 pm: eat your second meal with protein, carbohydrates, and fats
- After you eat your food drink your magnesium (before 5 pm)
- 9 pm drink your bulletproof coffee with collagen
- If collagen is powder put it inside coffee. If they are on pills drink them before coffee.
- After the bulletproof coffee, you can only drink water until the next day
- 30-minute simple exercise

DAY 9:

- 7 am: drink apple cider vinegar tea
- Wait for 30 minutes
- 7:30 drink morning coffee
- 11:00: pm eat your first meal with protein, carbohydrates, and fats
- Soon after that drink your potassium, b12, and biotin
- 4 pm: eat your second meal with protein, carbohydrates, and fats

- After you eat your food drink your magnesium (before 5 pm)
- 9 pm drink your bulletproof coffee with collagen
- If collagen is powder put it inside coffee. If they are on pills drink them before coffee.
- After the bulletproof coffee, you can only drink water until the next day
- 30-minute simple exercise

Day 10:

- 7 am: drink apple cider vinegar tea
- Wait for 30 minutes
- 7:30 drink morning coffee
- 11:00: pm eat your first meal with protein, carbohydrates, and fats
- Soon after that drink your potassium, b12, and biotin
- 4 pm: eat your second meal with protein, carbohydrates, and fats
- After you eat your food drink your magnesium (before 5 pm)
- 9 pm drink your bulletproof coffee with collagen
- If collagen is powder put it inside coffee. If they are on pills drink them before coffee.

- After the bulletproof coffee, you can only drink water until the next day
- 30-minute simple exercise

IN THE NEXT CHAPTER, I will tell you the changes for the next 10 days. I am very proud of you!

DAYS 11-20

*S*o happy you made it to day 11! This means you are very well committed to having the best health and body ever. Not many people make it to day 11 since it is hard for them to stop bad habits and start new ones. You should give yourself a pat on the back for your commitment and consistency. Those two, together, will give you results.

So these next 10 days I want you to do something. It will probably be hard for you if you are not used to it, it might not. But think about it, you already took sugar out of your diet, I think everything else after that will be easier. So here we go...

These next 10 days you will NOT be eating red meat. So keep your red meats in the freezer since you will not need them. Yes, you can eat everything else on the animal protein list in chapter 1 except red meat. These next 10 days will give your body some rest from that.

The first 10 days were a fast of 14/10 (14 hours fasting 10 hours of eating period). Now, for these next 10 days, you will increase your fasting to 16/8 (16 hours fasting 8 hours eating period). Don't worry, you will feel great. Remember to take your supplements because these will help you get the nutrients you need to feel good.

The time given on each day is an example. You can adjust the eating times depending on what time you wake up and go to bed. Just make sure you are fasting for 16 hours straight and a period of 8 hours (only) to eat. Make sure you are only drinking water the times you are fasting.

DAY 11:

- *remember No red meat
- 7 am: drink apple cider vinegar tea
- Wait for 30 minutes
- 7:30 am- drink morning coffee
- 12:00 pm- eat your first meal with protein, carbohydrates, and fats
- Soon after that, drink your potassium, b12, and biotin
- 4 pm- eat your second meal with protein, carbohydrates, and fats
- After you eat your food drink your magnesium
- 8 pm- drink your bulletproof coffee with collagen

- If collagen is powder put it inside coffee. If they are on pills drink them before coffee
- *after your coffee, the only thing you can put in your body is water until the next day
- 30-minute simple exercise

Day 12:

- *remember No red meat
- 7 am: drink apple cider vinegar tea
- Wait for 30 minutes
- 7:30 am- drink morning coffee
- 12:00 pm- eat your first meal with protein, carbohydrates, and fats
- Soon after that, drink your potassium, b12, and biotin
- 4 pm- eat your second meal with protein, carbohydrates, and fats
- After you eat your food drink your magnesium
- 8 pm- drink your bulletproof coffee with collagen
- If collagen is powder put it inside coffee. If they are on pills drink them before coffee
- *after your coffee, the only thing you can put in your body is water until the next day
- 30-minute simple exercise

DAY 13:

- *remember No red meat
- 7 am: drink apple cider vinegar tea
- Wait for 30 minutes
- 7:30 am- drink morning coffee
- 12:00 pm- eat your first meal with protein, carbohydrates, and fats
- Soon after that, drink your potassium, b12, and biotin
- 4 pm- eat your second meal with protein, carbohydrates, and fats
- After you eat your food drink your magnesium
- 8 pm- drink your bulletproof coffee with collagen
- If collagen is powder put it inside coffee. If they are on pills drink them before coffee
- *after your coffee, the only thing you can put in your body is water until the next day
- 30-minute simple exercise

DAY 14:

- *remember No red meat

- 7 am: drink apple cider vinegar tea
- Wait for 30 minutes
- 7:30 am- drink morning coffee
- 12:00 pm- eat your first meal with protein, carbohydrates, and fats
- Soon after that, drink your potassium, b12, and biotin
- 4 pm- eat your second meal with protein, carbohydrates, and fats
- After you eat your food drink your magnesium
- 8 pm- drink your bulletproof coffee with collagen
- If collagen is powder put it inside coffee. If they are on pills drink them before coffee
- *after your coffee, the only thing you can put in your body is water until the next day
- 30-minute simple exercise

DAY 15:

- *remember No red meat
- 7 am: drink apple cider vinegar tea
- Wait for 30 minutes
- 7:30 am- drink morning coffee
- 12:00 pm- eat your first meal with protein, carbohydrates, and fats

- Soon after that, drink your potassium, b12, and biotin
- 4 pm- eat your second meal with protein, carbohydrates, and fats
- After you eat your food drink your magnesium
- 8 pm- drink your bulletproof coffee with co

DAYS 21-30

*I*sn't this amazing or what? You made it through the first 20 days! This means you are capable of doing things you never thought you could do before.

So these next 10 days will be a little different. You will do an 18/6 intermittent fasting. This means you will fast for 18 hours and eat in between 6 hours period. Don't worry I think you will have a great time doing this. The times I show in every day are just examples so you can see how a day goes but you can adjust it to your schedule depending on what time you wake up in the day and what time you go to bed. Adjust it accordingly with 18 hours of fasting to 6 hours of eating period.

Now, good news, you can start eating red meats again. Bad news: these 10 days you will not consume any dairy. This means no cheese, half and half, butter, heavy cream, sour cream- nothing that comes from milk. So you may be asking, how can you keep the chicken from sticking to the pan without the butter? Simple, use olive oil, coconut oil, and avocado oil but nothing else.

These 10 days incorporate nuts as fat in both of your meals. I want you to get used to including these and eating them. I don't want you to only think about cheese as a only source of fat. Nuts are rich in nutrients.

One important thing you should know about fasting for 18 hours is the benefits for your body. Besides losing weight it also helps regenerate your cells. That means it will help you live longer and look younger. Now that you have fasted for 14 and 16 hours, you will find that fasting for 18 hours will be very easy and you will not feel hungry. Plus when you see those pounds start melting off, especially when your clothes start fitting big, you will feel more motivated

The Bulletproof coffee you will prepare these next 10 days will be different from the one you are used to making. If you don't feel hungry for this bullet proof coffee you don't have to drink it. You will probably fill full from your second meal. If you feel this way skip it and start your fast, drink your collagen with your second food. If you feel like drinking it, this is what you will need:

- 1 cup of brewed coffee (plain, no flavor)
- 1 tbsp of MCT oil
- 2 tbsp of almond milk
- collagen powder

How to prepare it:

Blend all ingredients together in a blender. Blend and serve in a mug. So are you ready to continue transforming your body these coming 10 days? Well, let's get started.

Day 21:

- *remember no dairy
- include nuts as a fat in your meals
- 7:00 am- drink apple cider vinegar tea
- Wait for 30 minutes
- 7:30 am- drink morning coffee
- 12:00 pm- eat your first meal with protein, carbohydrates, and fats
- Soon after that drink your potassium, b12, and biotin
- 4 pm- eat your second meal with protein, carbohydrates, and fats
- After you eat your food, drink your magnesium
- 6:00 pm- drink your bulletproof coffee without dairy (see above for recipe) with collagen
- If collagen is powder put it inside coffee. If they are on pills drink them before coffee
- *after you drink this, the only thing you can put in your body is water until the next day
- 30-minute simple exercise

DAY 22:

- *remember no dairy
- include nuts as a fat in your meals 7:00 am- drink apple cider vinegar tea
- Wait for 30 minutes
- 7:30 am- drink morning coffee
- 12:00 pm- eat your first meal with protein, carbohydrates, and fats
- Soon after that drink your potassium, b12, and biotin
- 3 pm- eat your second meal with protein, carbohydrates, and fats
- After you eat your food, drink your magnesium
- 6:00 pm- drink your bulletproof coffee without dairy (see above for recipe) with collagen
- If collagen is powder put it inside coffee. If they are on pills drink them before coffee
- *after you drink this, the only thing you can put in your body is water until the next day
- 30-minute simple exercise

DAY 23:

- *remember no dairy
- include nuts as a fat in your meals 7:00 am- drink apple cider vinegar tea

- Wait for 30 minutes
- 7:30 am- drink morning coffee
- 12:00 pm- eat your first meal with protein, carbohydrates, and fats
- Soon after that drink your potassium, b12, and biotin
- 3 pm- eat your second meal with protein, carbohydrates, and fats
- After you eat your food, drink your magnesium
- 6:00 pm- drink your bulletproof coffee without dairy (see above for recipe) with collagen
- If collagen is powder put it inside coffee. If they are on pills drink them before coffee
- *after you drink this, the only thing you can put in your body is water until the next day
- 30-minute simple exercise

DAY 24:

- *remember no dairy
- include nuts as a fat in your meals 7:00 am- drink apple cider vinegar tea
- Wait for 30 minutes
- 7:30 am- drink morning coffee
- 12:00 pm- eat your first meal with protein, carbohydrates, and fats

- Soon after that drink your potassium, b12, and biotin
- 3 pm- eat your second meal with protein, carbohydrates, and fats
- After you eat your food, drink your magnesium
- 6:00 pm- drink your bulletproof coffee without dairy (see above for recipe) with collagen
- If collagen is powder put it inside coffee. If they are on pills drink them before coffee
- *after you drink this, the only thing you can put in your body is water until the next day
- 30-minute simple exercise

Day 25:

- *remember no dairy
- include nuts as a fat in your meals 7:00 am- drink apple cider vinegar tea
- Wait for 30 minutes
- 7:30 am- drink morning coffee
- 12:00 pm- eat your first meal with protein, carbohydrates, and fats
- Soon after that drink your potassium, b12, and biotin
- 3 pm- eat your second meal with protein, carbohydrates, and fats
- After you eat your food, drink your magnesium

- 6:00 pm- drink your bulletproof coffee without dairy (see above for recipe) with collagen
- If collagen is powder put it inside coffee. If they are on pills drink them before coffee
- *after you drink this, the only thing you can put in your body is water until the next day
- 30-minute simple exercise

Day 26:

- *remember no dairy
- include nuts as a fat in your meals
- 7:00 am- drink apple cider vinegar tea
- Wait for 30 minutes
- 7:30 am- drink morning coffee
- 12:00 pm- eat your first meal with protein, carbohydrates, and fats
- Soon after that drink your potassium, b12, and biotin
- 3 pm- eat your second meal with protein, carbohydrates, and fats
- After you eat your food, drink your magnesium
- 6:00 pm- drink your bulletproof coffee without dairy (see above for recipe) with collagen
- If collagen is powder put it inside coffee. If they are on pills drink them before coffee

- *after you drink this, the only thing you can put in your body is water until the next day
- 30-minute simple exercise

DAY 27:

- *remember no dairy
- include nuts as a fat in your meals
- 7:00 am- drink apple cider vinegar tea
- Wait for 30 minutes
- 7:30 am- drink morning coffee
- 12:00 pm- eat your first meal with protein, carbohydrates, and fats
- Soon after that drink your potassium, b12, and biotin
- 3 pm- eat your second meal with protein, carbohydrates, and fats
- After you eat your food, drink your magnesium
- 6:00 pm- drink your bulletproof coffee without dairy (see above for recipe) with collagen
- If collagen is powder put it inside coffee. If they are on pills drink them before coffee
- *after you drink this, the only thing you can put in your body is water until the next day
- 30-minute simple exercise

DAY 28:

- *remember no dairy
- include nuts as a fat in your meals
- 7:00 am- drink apple cider vinegar tea
- Wait for 30 minutes
- 7:30 am- drink morning coffee
- 12:00 pm- eat your first meal with protein, carbohydrates, and fats
- Soon after that drink your potassium, b12, and biotin
- 3 pm- eat your second meal with protein, carbohydrates, and fats
- After you eat your food, drink your magnesium
- 6:00 pm- drink your bulletproof coffee without dairy (see above for recipe) with collagen
- If collagen is powder put it inside coffee. If they are on pills drink them before coffee
- *after you drink this, the only thing you can put in your body is water until the next day
- 30-minute simple exercise

DAY 29:

- *remember no dairy
- include nuts as a fat in your meals
- 7:00 am- drink apple cider vinegar tea

- Wait for 30 minutes
- 7:30 am- drink morning coffee
- 12:00 pm- eat your first meal with protein, carbohydrates, and fats
- Soon after that drink your potassium, b12, and biotin
- 3 pm- eat your second meal with protein, carbohydrates, and fats
- After you eat your food, drink your magnesium
- 6:00 pm- drink your bulletproof coffee without dairy (see above for recipe) with collagen
- If collagen is powder put it inside coffee. If they are on pills drink them before coffee
- *after you drink this, the only thing you can put in your body is water until the next day
- 30-minute simple exercise

DAY 30:

- *remember no dairy
- include nuts as a fat in your meals
- 7:00 am- drink apple cider vinegar tea
- Wait for 30 minutes
- 7:30 am- drink morning coffee
- 12:00 pm- eat your first meal with protein, carbohydrates, and fats

- Soon after that drink your potassium, b12, and biotin
- 3 pm- eat your second meal with protein, carbohydrates, and fats
- After you eat your food, drink your magnesium
- 6:00 pm- drink your bulletproof coffee without dairy (see above for recipe) with collagen
- If collagen is powder put it inside coffee. If they are on pills drink them before coffee
- *after you drink this, the only thing you can put in your body is water until the next day
- 30-minute simple exercise

ON THIS DAY in the morning, you will weigh yourself and do body measurements. You will measure your bust, waist, right and left biceps, hips, right and left thighs. With these measurements, you will compare from the first day when you started. Write your final weight and measurements below.

DATE:_____
   Ending weight:_____

BODY MEASUREMENTS:

. . .

BICEPS L/R:_____

    Bust:_____

    Waist:_____

    Hip: _____

    Thighs L/R:_____

I DON'T USE weight as the only thing to measure my progress because it always fluctuates. The body measurements are more accurate plus you can tell when the jeans are fitting bigger on you.

IF YOU GOT to this last day, you are awesome!!!! That means you have broken old habits an put on new habits. You should be proud of yourself. I am proud of you because you did it!

MAINTENANCE PHASE

$\mathcal{L}$et me tell you there is good news once you have achieved your desired healthy weight. So I will put them in detail for you. Remember You will not go back to your old ways or old habits. This is to maintain your weight. So to maintain your weight means you won't do everything you were doing before. So Fasting time will be shorter and you can add some fruits to your diet. So here we go.

Monitor your weight weekly

Like I said before, your weight fluctuates. I say if it's 3 lbs up or down it's okay. Remember sometimes we retain water and that could be why. Don't get scared. It is better if you monitor how your clothes are fitting that's a more accurate way of knowing you are going up or down in weight. If they fit like it is supposed to then you are maintaining your weight, but if it's getting tighter then you should pay more attention to how you are eating.

ACV tea

You can continue to drink the morning tea with apple cider vinegar and lemon. It will help to alkalinize your body.

No MCT Oil

Since you won't be doing long periods of fasting, you won't need the MCT oil if you don't want to.

Decrease fasting times

Since you don't need to lose any more weight, you won't need to fast as often. Maybe instead of doing 18/6, you can do 14/10 or 12/12

More fats and protein

You need to incorporate more fat and protein. That fat will be used more for energy and continue to burn fat. And you will need the protein to build muscle.

Eat fruits

If fruits and vegetables are very important to losing weight, they are also important so you can keep the weight. For this, eat only 5 pieces of fruit or vegetables a day and you will see you will not go up in weight. You will eat ONLY berry fruits. These are not high in sugars.

Root vegetables

You can include root vegetables. These are good carbs. So if you eat this, you will have to reduce your regular vegetable portion to ½ cup and ½ cup of root vegetables.

Supplements

Yes, continue consuming the supplements. These help us with our muscles, hormones, articulations, and collagen.

Exercise

Yes, you have to continue exercising. This is a must to maintain your weight. A 91% of the people that maintain their weight do exercise.

Sleep Well

Sleep what you need. Who would have thought that sleeping well can reduce your waist size?. Yes, it is true. Not enough sleep will make you hungry.

Control Stress

Stress can cause you to have cravings. This will make you look for junk food instead of the healthy foods you should be eating.

So this is how you maintain your weight when reaching your goal weight. It will be way easier since all the hard stuff you had already done.

CONCLUSION

$\mathcal{T}$here are no words to describe how proud I am of you for completing this challenge. Even though this is a short book, I am sure you learned so much. Use this knowledge to teach other people about good health and longevity. Many people need guidance these days. They will thank you!

ONCE YOU ARE DONE with the challenge. Start it over again and over again until you have reached your desired weight. Make sure you follow it correctly and you will see that muffing top gets shredded quickly. When you reach your desired weight, go to the maintenance phase and continue exercising.

. . .

YOU WILL GET USED to this new lifestyle and all the temptations you had before will be gone forever.

IF YOU LOVED THIS BOOK. Make sure you leave a review on amazon. Reviews don't come easy, but when they do, they have a big impact. Thank you so much.

REFERENCES

*H*ealth Essentials. (2022, March 3). *Intermittent fasting: How it works and 4 types explained.* Retrieved February 6, 2022, from https://health. clevelandclinic.org/intermittent-fasting-4-different-types-explained/

Leal, D. (2021, June 30). *Why eating fat makes you healthy.* Https://Www.Verywellfit.Com/Why-Eating-Fat-Keeps-You-Healthy-3121407. Retrieved June 2, 2022, from https://www.verywellfit.com/why-eating-fat-keeps-you-healthy-3121407

Times of India. (2021, April 13). *Morning or night: What's a better time to have apple cider vinegar?* Https://Timesofindia.Indiatimes.Com/Life-Style/Health-Fitness/Diet/Morning-or-Night-Whats-a-Better-Time-to-Have-Apple-Cider-Vinegar/Photosto-ry/81469993.Cms. Retrieved June 2, 2022, from https://

timesofindia.indiatimes.com/life-style/health-fitness/
diet/morning-or-night-whats-a-better-time-to-have-
apple-cider-vinegar/photostory/81469993.cms

Fung, D. J. (2016). *The obesity code: Unlocking the Secrets of Weightloss*. Audible studio.